Instant

chakra healing

Exercises and guidance for everyday wellness

JENNIE HARDING

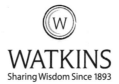

WATKINS

Sharing Wisdom Since 1893

Instant Chakra Healing
Jennie Harding

This edition published in the UK and USA in
2018 by Watkins,
an imprint of Watkins Media Limited
19 Cecil Court
London WC2N 4EZ

First published in 2006 by Duncan Baird
Publishers Ltd as *Live Better: Chakra Therapy*

enquiries@watkinspublishing.com

Managing Editors: Grace Cheetham and
    Daniel Hurst
Editor: Rebecca Miles
Designers: Georgina Hewitt and
    Glen Wilkins
Production: Uzma Taj
Model Photography: Matthew Ward
Commissioned artwork: Glen Wilkins

A CIP record for this book is available from
the British Library

ISBN: 978-1-84899-254-2

10 9 8 7 6 5 4 3 2 1

Typeset in Palatino
Colour reproduction by XY Digital
Printed in China

Notes:
Abbreviations used throughout this book:
CE Common Era (the equivalent of AD)
BCE Before the Common Era (the equivalent
of BC)
b. born, d. died

www.watkinspublishing.com

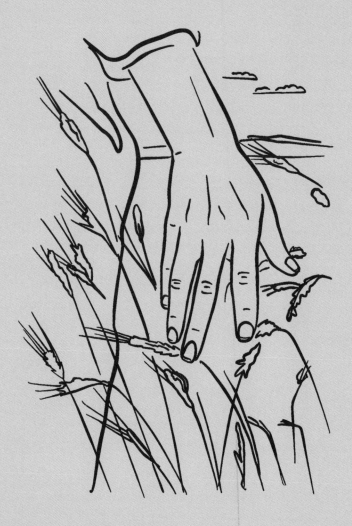

Contents

INTRODUCTION

Welcome to this guide to enhanced relaxation and well-being, based around the system of the chakras that originate from India. This is a philosophy that shows us how to live in an inspired and harmonious way by gaining an in-depth understanding of the energy framework of the body.

Living as we do in a fast-paced world, we tend to focus our attention on the physical aspects of existence – the things we can see and touch. For example, we know that a chair exists because we can see it, feel it and sit on it. Thousands of physical perceptions fill our minds every day and sometimes these can become a blur.

Ancient Indian teachings share a different concept of life. Besides physical experience, there is a belief in an underlying system that is invisible, but permeates all things. It consists of energy called prana, meaning "life force" or "vital energy". This energy enters the body at different frequencies via a series of special sites or energy centres, each one called a chakra; this word means "wheel" in the ancient Indian language Sanskrit.

The chakra system is part of the tradition of yoga, which began in India several thousand years ago. Indian sages regarded the chakras as the means whereby universal energy, the force that creates all things, is stepped down in frequency so that the human body can use it. One of the fundamental ancient universal laws is that energy precedes form – in modern times aspects of quantum physics express this same idea. So as well as having a physical body that we can see and touch, we also have an invisible "energy body" that permeates our solid structure. The chakras are our energy blueprint, needed in the invisible realm to create, heal and balance the human body in the physical realm.

There are seven major chakras in the human body, and this book will enable you to discover what and where they are and how working, balancing and supporting them can enhance your life. Making this journey will unlock the positive effects of chakra energy in your body. Once you open up to this, your perception of life will develop in new and enriching ways.

CHAPTER

Chakra Basics

A chakra is a place in the body where energy spins in a vortex. It is sometimes described as having petals, like a lotus flower; when the chakra is open, and its energy is flowing freely, the petals are spread out, and when it is closed, depleted or blocked, the petals are tightly shut. This image is often used in visualizations to help open and maintain the flow of life-giving energy through all seven chakras, and we will be practising techniques that support this later in the book.

Each chakra is located both at the front and back of the body, passing through the three-dimensional structure of the physical frame. For example, there is a location in the middle of the chest area called the Heart Chakra, which spins into the body, through the spine and out between the shoulder blades. Each of the seven major chakras has a front and back aspect, though as you will see in the diagram on page 10, only one side tends to be shown.

The word "chakra" is also linguistically close to Sanskrit terms for the cosmos, or the universe, and the chakra system is one illustration of how we form part of the universe, and the universe forms part of us. We come from energy, we take physical form, we journey through life and we return to energy; this is the pattern of existence.

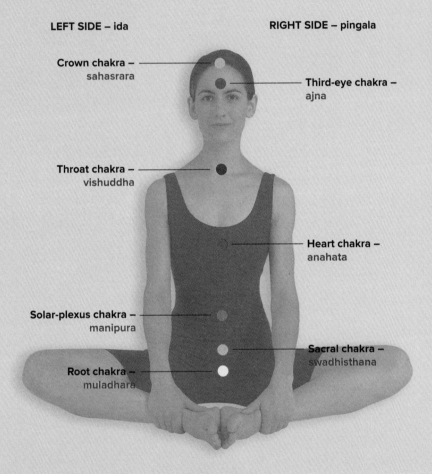

LEFT SIDE – ida

RIGHT SIDE – pingala

Crown chakra –
sahasrara

Third-eye chakra –
ajna

Throat chakra –
vishuddha

Heart chakra –
anahata

Solar-plexus chakra –
manipura

Sacral chakra –
swadhisthana

Root chakra –
muladhara

Centre – sushumna

LOCATING THE CHAKRAS

The seven major chakras are located from the crown of the head, down through the forehead, throat, chest and abdomen, to the base of the spine. Indian tradition also mentions minor chakras, for example in the palms of the hands, but the seven major chakras are the most important. They are like transformers on an electrical grid, where the current changes in frequency.

Each of the seven major chakras has an associated colour – together making up the full rainbow spectrum. The root and sacral chakras are red and orange – warm colours to denote the chakras' links to physical energy. The solar plexus is golden yellow, full of dynamism. The heart is green, vibrant and expansive like growing plants; and the throat, third eye and crown centres have blue and purple hues, linked to the cool but fast vibrations of the energies of communication, thought and creativity. Each chakra is related to different types of daily activity. We use our chakra energies all the time; by learning more about chakras we can do so consciously.

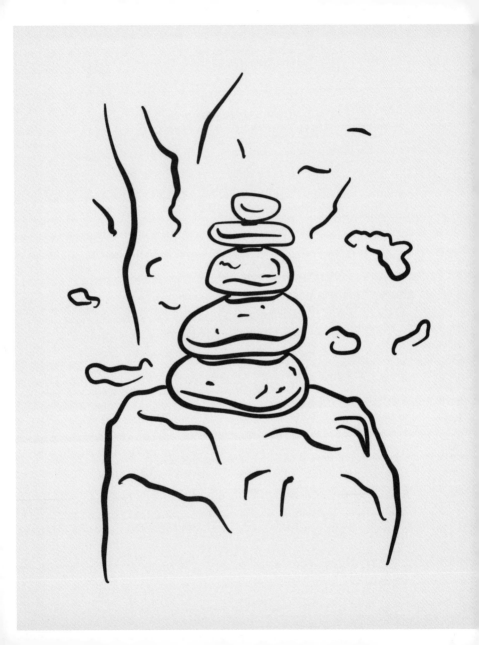

The best and safest thing is to keep a balance in your life, acknowledge the great powers around us and in us. If you can do that, and live that way, you are really a wise man.

EURIPIDES
(C.484–C.406BCE)

HOW CAN THE CHAKRAS HELP ME?

Learning more about the types of energy within you, where they are concentrated and how they relate to your feelings or moods, can make a huge difference to the way you deal with the everyday demands of life. Instead of reacting to situations in ways that arise from stress, resentment or pressure, you will be able to re-interpret what is happening to you and use chakra-based tools to help you cope.

Your chakra energies can be influenced in many ways, for example through simple exercises, visualizations, the use of essential oils or crystals, or the postures of yoga – all of which you will find later in this book. Once you learn to locate your chakras, understand a little about their relationships to your physical body, and experience their benefits to your energy body, you will begin to understand yourself better, creating a heightened state of awareness. This allows you to observe what happens to you in life without being immediately sucked in and emotionally drained by your experiences.

We all go through times when we feel as though life is getting on top of us. Working with the chakra system helps us to identify why we are feeling a certain way, and teaches us to pause, feel changes in our bodies, and react differently to whatever confronts us.

If you pay attention to and support your chakras, you will help to optimize the energy flow around your body. In turn, the cleansing, unblocking and rebalancing of your chakra energies, usually in a progression from the root to the crown, works as part of a holistic approach to well-being that positively affects all aspects of the mind, body and spirit. Each chakra operates on a different frequency, but they are all linked. These frequencies also equate to, and influence, different states of mind or activity with which we engage every day. We explore the various physical, emotional and psychological links between our bodies and each of the chakras in detail in Chapters Two and Three. From this you will be able to identify which of your chakras may need particular work, in terms of rebalancing and support, in order to improve certain symptoms you may be experiencing.

THE CIRCLE OF LIFE

Change is a constant factor in life. It is, however, something we often find difficult. We don't like things to change, we feel safer if we think things will not change, and we can become upset or depressed when external factors show us that actually change is inevitable.

The natural world is a great teacher of change, and yet in the developed nations we are becoming increasingly cut off from it. The cycles of the seasons and the way in which plants, birds and other creatures react to the environment are far distant from lives spent in buildings of concrete, steel, glass and plastic, or travelling in metal cars, trains or planes. We think we can control all aspects of existence, and yet deep down many people feel empty, or even as though their lives are out of control.

We need to reconnect with the idea that energy, the dynamic force that creates the universe, is constantly in motion. Stars, planets, even galaxies are born, rise to brilliance, fade or perhaps explode into particles that spin and begin to reform new systems – there is life, death and then rebirth. This idea is deeply embedded in the philosophy and spiritual beliefs of India. We experience these cycles constantly throughout the journey of life in the physical plane, but we come from energy and eventually we will return to that state.

Through the chakra frequencies, we can experience the dynamism of universal energy in the body itself. As we move from the inspirational level of the crown, to the intuitive knowing of the third eye, to the voice at the throat giving sound and meaning to ideas, to the feelings in the heart and the confidence in the solar plexus, to reach out to other people at the sacrum and take action at the root, we trigger new cycles of thoughts, feelings and actions – and so life moves forward.

Understanding the chakras will help you to accept change. Knowing that your energies move and fluctuate constantly makes change exciting. Life is a dynamic, creative and evolving journey, not static and linear, but three-dimensional, colourful and vibrant. We are here to experience the world joyfully with open hearts and minds – in full awareness. All we have to do is allow it.

USING THIS BOOK

This book is designed to help you to be aware of your chakra centres in your everyday life, so that you can balance your own energies and live more harmoniously, within your own body and in the world around you. Different kinds of exercises and visualizations will enable you to explore your own energy levels and maintain balance of body, mind and spirit.

In Chapter Two we see how the chakras relate to the physical body by finding out exactly where these energy centres are, and how they link to our physical sense of well-being. Try out the practical tasks designed to help you move through energy blocks and revitalize yourself.

In Chapter Three we will explore each chakra in detail, so you can develop your understanding of each of the seven energy centres in turn. We learn about the colour vibration of each chakra and its significance; then discover the links between that centre and different physical, emotional or mental states. Making this connection helps you to understand your moods better and to influence them positively. Discover how to rebalance each chakra with a special yoga posture, and explore it in depth using a unique visualization designed to harmonize the energy in that area.

Chapter Four introduces ways of working with all seven chakras collectively as a total energy system, through visualization, and use of sound, fragrances and crystals, to rebalance your whole chakra system.

To get the best from this book, I suggest that you read it through once to explore all aspects of the c hakras. You will find that certain chakras feel of more relevance to you than others. Note which these are, then return to their specific sections to work on them first. Choose a couple of the suggested balancing techniques and start to practise them once a day for a few days. Notice any effects in the chakra area you have chosen, for example more energy, a sense of vitality, or an easing of mood. Changes may be subtle, or you may feel a marked sense of renewal. As you revitalize one chakra, you may find yourself drawn to work on others, in an upward spiral of the support, balance and harmony of your body's energy.

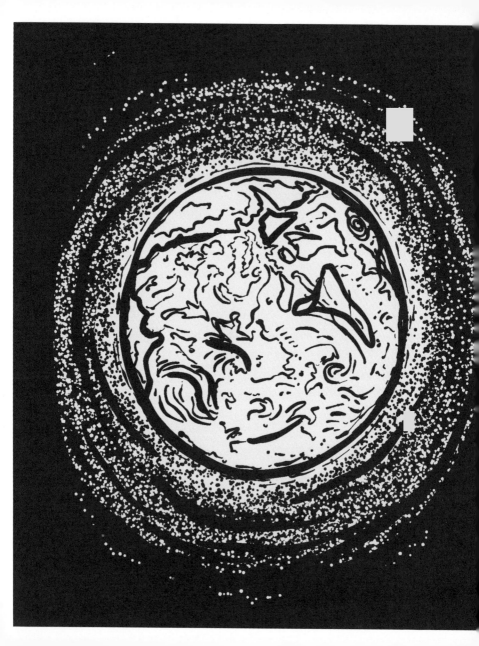

In everything that moves through the universe, I see my own body, and in everything that governs the universe, my own soul.

CHANG TSAI
(1021–1077)

CHAPTER

Chakras and the Body

Although the chakras are part of an invisible energetic framework for the body, they are also connected to the physical anatomy. In this chapter we explore this relationship more closely, showing how to locate and identify chakra issues that link to health and vitality.

Illness is sometimes called a state of "dis-ease" – a lack of ease, or relaxation, in the system. Stress, whether emotional, physical or mental, is a major cause of imbalance. It is the factor that impedes the flow of chakra energy, and, over time, may manifest itself as physical imbalances in the body. Remember, energy precedes form; whatever appears physically

TWO...

has its roots in something energetic that has fallen out of balance. Gently working to restore the appropriate chakra frequency helps the body's powerful self-healing mechanisms to restore harmony.

It is important to emphasize that chakra work is not designed to diagnose medical illness. If you feel at all concerned about your health, consult a doctor. If a medical condition occurs it may have arisen because of an earlier energy imbalance of some kind, but, at this stage, it may require more direct intervention. However, working with your chakras does help to maintain everyday balance in your system and to prevent chronic, mild or long term health issues that can affect the general pattern of your life.

HOW CHAKRAS BALANCE THE BODY

One of the key ways chakras influence the physical body is via the hormone system. The seven major chakras are all connected to glands or organs responsible for different hormonal activities. Hormones are chemicals that transmit instructions around the body. They are a vital yet subtle element of body chemistry, possibly the closest aspect of the human form to the energy body itself, and are said to be directly influenced by chakra energies.

Chakra work can help to keep the body's hormonal activity in balance. Whether you choose a physical task (such as a yoga posture), a mental visualization or another approach, you will be helping to maintain the delicate inner balance of the associated hormones.

The root chakra is linked to the adrenal glands, which produce hormones associated with the "fight or flight" response and our survival instinct. The sacrum chakra links to the ovaries and testes, which produce sex hormones. The solar plexus chakra connects to the pancreas, which produces insulin. The heart chakra is linked to the thymus, a key player in our immune system. The throat chakra is connected to the thyroid, which releases hormones important for cellular growth and repair. The third eye chakra is linked to the pituitary gland at the base of the brain, which directs the activity of many of the body's hormones; and the crown chakra is linked to the pineal gland, which releases melatonin, and governs our responses to dark and light.

To cleanse and balance all chakra areas, and promote a corresponding harmonizing effect on your hormones, try this exercise. Sit comfortably in a chair with arms and legs uncrossed. Close your eyes, relax and breathe regularly. Starting at the crown of the head, visualize a flow of white light passing into the head, then slowly travelling down the front of your body, through the third eye, throat, heart, solar plexus, sacral and root areas. When you reach the base of the spine, imagine the light travelling up your back, from the root up through all the chakra areas to the crown of the head. Visualize this oval shape of white light running around your body in this circuit for a few minutes, as you breathe calmly.

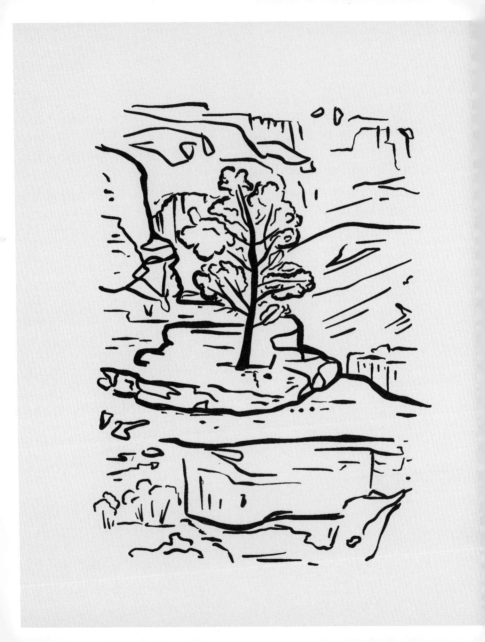

Be still like a mountain, flow like a great river.

LAO-TZU
(C.604–C.531BCE)

THE ROOT AND SACRAL CHAKRAS AND THE BODY

Starting with the root and sacral chakras, the next few pages explore physical links between the chakras and the body. These ideas will help you to better interpret and understand your body. I also suggest ways to support and rebalance your system to promote optimum health.

The root chakra

The main physical location of the root chakra is at the base of the spine. This area is often prone to injury and strain through heavy lifting, and persistent weakness in the lower back suggests that the root chakra may need strengthening. A simple way to do this is to use vetiver essential oil (*Vetiveria zizanoides*), which energizes the root chakra. Add 2 drops to a bath, or blend 2 drops in one tsp/5ml of vegetable carrier oil and massage into the lower back for a warming and invigorating effect.

This chakra is also closely linked to the kidneys and adrenal glands. The adrenals can be affected by stress;

immune conditions such as chronic fatigue syndrome may be caused by adrenal overload. If you feel that stress affects your immunity, perhaps making you susceptible to frequent colds or flu, try the root chakra support techniques on pages 38–47 to strengthen your system.

The sacral chakra

The sacral chakra is linked to the male and female sex organs. It is especially vulnerable in women, being connected to the hormonal shifts of the menstrual cycle as well as to major bodily changes such as pregnancy or the menopause. Irregular menstruation, heavy periods or PMS all indicate that this chakra needs energizing. A key essential oil in sacral chakra care is sandalwood (*Santalum album*); it is a tonic and helps to strengthen the sex organs. Women can add 3 drops to a daily bath for three days before the onset of a period to soothe the area and re-energize this chakra.

Sacral chakra energy is also linked to large intestine function. If you suffer from conditions such as constipation or irregular bowel rhythm, you will benefit from practising the Cat yoga posture on pages 54–55.

THE SOLAR PLEXUS AND HEART CHAKRAS AND THE BODY

Both the solar plexus and heart chakras link to parts of the body that react powerfully to feelings. If we are afraid, "butterflies in the stomach" are a signal from the solar plexus; if we are upset, an emotion felt in the heart shows that the heart chakra is affected.

The solar plexus chakra

The physical location of this chakra is just under the rib cage, by the stomach, small intestine, liver, gallbladder, spleen and pancreas – all organs involved in digestive function. Signs of over-acidity, stomach cramps or poor digestion all call for solar plexus chakra work. The digestive system is highly susceptible to stress, and the physical solar plexus is a junction point in the nervous system that reacts to outside influences, often with deep-rooted feelings such as anger. Place both hands over the solar plexus and breathe deeply, counting ten breaths in and out, to help stablize and rebalance this chakra and calm the emotions and the digestive organs.

The heart chakra

The heart chakra is closely associated with the heart itself, although the chakra location is in the middle of the chest and the organ sits slightly to the left. If you ever experience any unusual symptoms such as tingling or pains in the chest you must be medically examined as soon as possible; these could be signs of acute heart dysfunction. If you suffer from high blood pressure, the heart chakra tools on pages 68–77 will be of help to you – they balance your heart chakra, which in turn supports a healthy circulatory system. Also, place your hands directly over your heart chakra and breathe slowly and regularly to relax this area and ease stress.

The heart chakra is also linked to the thymus gland higher up the chest, which produces cells vital to immune system function. Support the heart chakra and thymus with cardamom essential oil (*Elettaria cardamomum*). Blend 2 drops with one tsp/5ml of vegetable carrier oil, and massage daily into the upper chest, especially during the winter. This can help prevent viral infections such as colds or flu, and also soothes coughs.

THE THROAT AND THIRD EYE CHAKRAS AND THE BODY

When we reach the throat and third eye chakra areas we are moving away from the purely physical bodily associations between the lower chakras and the body, and into the realms of speech, thoughts and mental activity.

The throat chakra

The throat chakra sits in the middle of the collar bone area, over the voice box. Its energy can be diminished by over use of the voice; however, it can be energized by toning particular sacred sounds (see pp.114–115).

This area is prone to infections because of its proximity to bacteria breathed in from outside the body. Manuka essential oil (*Leptospermum scoparium*) is an excellent throat chakra remedy; blend 2 drops in one tsp/5ml of vegetable carrier oil and massage into the throat area daily to ward off infections.

The throat chakra is also closely linked to the thyroid gland, which is located in the central throat area. Any over- or underactivity of the thyroid can be supported by using the throat chakra tools on pages 78–87. Working on the throat chakra can also help to balance the thyroid gland energetically. This is helpful if you are receiving medical treatment for any thyroid conditions.

The third eye chakra

The third eye chakra sits between the eyebrows, close to the bridge of the nose. The anatomical structures associated with the sense of smell are located behind this ridge of bone just inside the skull, and these link to areas deep within the brain. Any problems with the sense of smell, such as temporary loss, can be helped by using third eye chakra tools (see pp. 88–97). Essential oil of basil (*Ocimum basilicum*) in a vaporizer or diffuser (3 drops for up to an hour effect) clears the third eye chakra energy easily and also aids mental concentration.

Being close to the eyes also links this chakra to conditions such as eye strain, headaches and migraine. Support the chakra and these complaints by rubbing your palms together briskly, and placing them over your eyes for a few minutes to soothe and relax the whole area.

THE CROWN CHAKRA AND THE BODY

The crown chakra sits on the very top of the head, where the bones of the skull called the fontanelles join. These bones are not yet joined at birth but fuse together at the age of about 18 months. The crown chakra represents the highest energy frequency in the body, and as such is linked to mental and emotional conditions.

Low levels of crown chakra energy are associated with conditions such as depression. The chakra itself is linked to the pineal gland, which reacts to the amount of light or darkness, regulating our sleeping and waking cycles. In modern life, we spend far too much time in artificial light and not enough time in natural light, so our body's natural cycles are disrupted. This can lead to conditions such as SAD (Seasonal Affective Disorder) where the body reacts with depression to lack of light. A simple remedy for many mild depressive states, including PMS, is to walk outside in the middle of the day when the sun is at its highest for just 15 minutes. This greatly improves pineal function and also helps increase crown chakra energy. Strong daylight, even if the sun is not shining, will still be effective even in the winter months.

To maintain and harmonize the crown chakra it is important to get the balance right between the different frequencies of the various major chakras. A simple daily breathing exercise will help you achieve this. It works most efficiently if you have bare feet. To begin, stand straight with your feet shoulder width apart, arms by your sides. Relax and take a few deep breaths. Now focus your attention on the soles of your feet. Feel where they join the ground. Breathe in, and slowly raise your arms above your head; feel the lightness of the energy there. Breathe out, and lower your arms, bringing your focus back down to your feet. Repeat three times. Then stand and relax, noticing how you feel.

Meditation is a practice that supports not just the crown chakra but all the chakras. It can be defined as relaxed contemplation, and can be experienced in many ways. Try concentrating for a few moments on a real or visualized candle flame. This brings stillness and inner peace, from the crown to the root chakra.

Chakra Profiles

In this chapter you will find a detailed profile of each chakra, along with many ideas, exercises, visualizations and tools for transformation. Now our journey into the chakra map deepens into thorough explorations of different aspects of each frequency level. It will guide you into yourself, so that you can work with chakra energies and experience their effects directly.

Chakra work is subtle, slow and unfolds at your own pace. As you read each profile, you will find that some chakras seem more relevant to you than others at this time. Trust your own perception. No-one else can tell you what is right for you; only you can decide what needs most help and where to begin. The more you return to the chakra profiles, the more you will find that your needs change; other chakras will become important, and you can work with these in turn.

Keep a notebook of your experiences. Consider what works for you and what doesn't, note your impressions, what you feel, and how your perceptions of yourself and your life change. Self-observation, self-awareness and self-realization are all part of chakra work as an ongoing process; you will become a more active and more sensitive participant in life, not just an onlooker. "Know thyself" is a saying that was carved over the entrance to the shrine of the ancient Greek oracle at Delphi; it still holds true today.

THE ROOT CHAKRA

Our journey through the chakras starts at the base of the spine where the root chakra glows a deep red. Its Sanskrit name, *muladhara*, means "root, or central support". Think of a tree, towering up to the sky. It can only stand so tall because it has a huge tap root, a deep anchor sunk into the ground supporting its upward growth. The root chakra is the frequency that anchors us and grounds us in physical existence; its element is earth.

Many of us are not grounded at all – we live our entire lives in our heads, preoccupied with the business – or the busy-ness – of mental distraction; the myriad sensations and external demands of the outside world. If you are the kind of person who suddenly notices a bruise on your leg and wonders how you got it, or you keep knocking yourself or dropping things, take note of these signs of lack of body awareness. You are not centred in your physical body, and your root chakra needs some energy.

Root chakra function is directly linked to adrenal gland activity as we have already seen. Adrenal reactions are set up in the body to get you into a state of alert to keep you alive. This is the "fight or flight" response. Root chakra energy is closely connected to physical survival. For all our beliefs in ourselves as a civilized species, regarding survival we still have the physiology of our cave man ancestors who often had to run for their lives. The problem with modern life is that it generates mental stress that keeps us in the "fight or flight" state for extended periods and does not allow us sufficient time to recover. This can cause adrenal overload, tiredness, exhaustion and general weakness. These are also signs of deficiency in root chakra energy.

When the root chakra is strong, there is a sense of stability in body and mind, a feeling of being centred and a trust in ones ability to cope with life. Root chakra energy gives you strength and well-being as well as a sense of being utterly at home in your own body. It also connects you powerfully with the earth. Take the opportunity as often as you can, weather permitting, to allow your bare feet to touch the ground. This is an extremely simple and effective root chakra tonic.

ROOT CHAKRA EMOTIONS

Because the root chakra is strongly associated with survival, it connects with deep-seated emotions of fear, insecurity and instability. Feelings of insecurity can make us lash out in impatience or anger at those around us because we hold them responsible for our instability. The truth is, we have to find that centre, that core of strength within ourselves. Nobody else can give it to us.

Persistent lower back problems can also be emotionally linked to this chakra. The spine is the body's central support; its base links to the hips, which help to move us forward. Lower back problems make us freeze up, causing immobility. This can be due to frozen or tense emotions. Working with the root chakra, and talking through any issues relating to lack of support or feeling emotionally blocked can open the chakra and help the back pain.

Once the root is re-energized, we feel strong again and able to deal with whatever confronts us. Positive root chakra energy creates open and balanced body language, ready to interact in life without judgement.

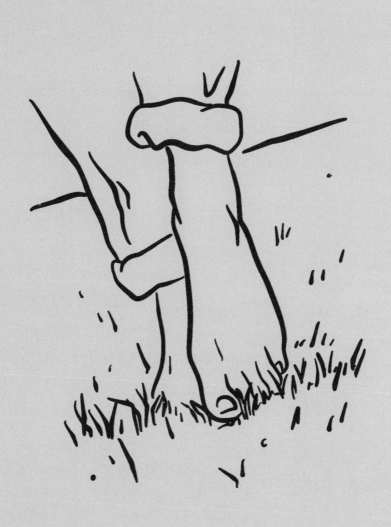

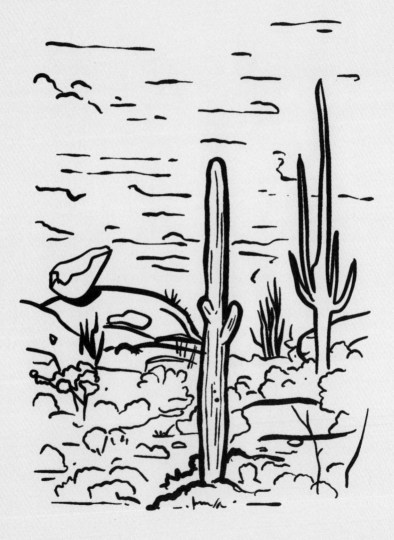

Nothing is rich but the inexhaustible wealth of nature. She shows us only surfaces, but she is a million fathoms deep.

RALPH WALDO EMERSON
(1803–1882)

ROOT CHAKRA YOGA

Yoga postures or asanas are part of the ancient system of Ayurveda – Indian traditional medicine that uses exercise, herbs, essential oils and massage to help rebalance the physical and energetic bodies. A simple yoga posture to support the root chakra is the Half Spinal Twist. This energizes the chakra as well as toning the digestive system. Only twist as far as you feel comfortable; your spine will loosen in time. Breathe regularly as you work.

1 Kneel down with your legs together and sit on your heels. Now shift so you are sitting to the left of your feet.

2 Lift your right leg over your left, and place your right foot close to the outside of the left knee. Keep your left heel close to your buttocks and sit up straight.

3 Place your left elbow on the outside of your right knee, and put your right arm on the floor behind your right buttock. Inhale, and as you exhale twist slowly as far as you can to the right, drawing the knee inward all the time.

4 Release the posture slowly, then repeat on the other side.

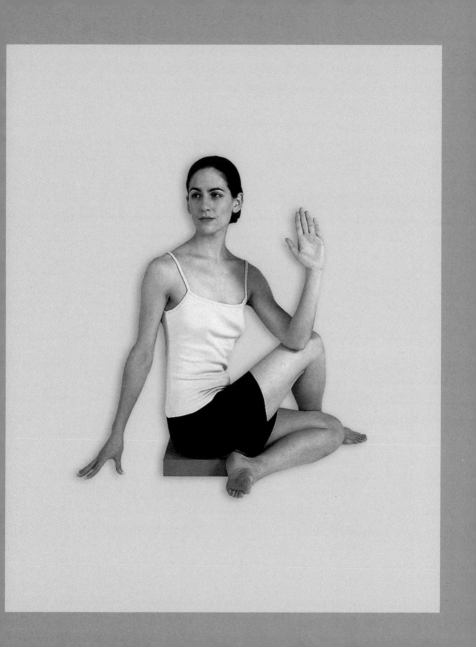

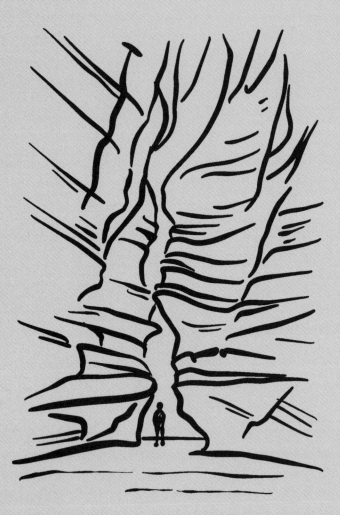

ROOT CHAKRA VISUALIZATION

Another way to re-energize the root chakra is to use the power of the mind by practising this visualization.

Find a quiet space to relax. Sit in a chair, legs uncrossed, hands in your lap. Take a few deep breaths. Focus attention on the base of your spine, the location of the root chakra. Notice any warmth, coolness or lack of feeling. Then imagine that from the base of your spine, a strong tap root is extending deep into the earth to the core of the planet. When your sense of this root is strong, breathe in, and as you inhale imagine deep red energy flooding upwards, spreading into your root chakra area as you exhale. This energy is warm, powerful and nourishing. Allow your root chakra to be bathed in this deep red colour; notice how you feel as you repeatedly breathe the energy up and spread it as you exhale.

To finish, imagine your tap root connection is being drawn back up from the earth to sit at the base of your spine again. Repeat this exercise whenever you need root chakra energy.

THE SACRAL CHAKRA

The Sacral chakra is known as *svadhisthana* in Sanskrit, meaning "your dwelling place". This phrase is subtle – who or what dwells there? The answer is that the sacral chakra is the home of your creativity. It is the creative impulse that ensures the survival of the human species, which is why the sacral chakra is also connected to human sexuality and the twofold aspects of male and female that combine together to create new life.

The colour of the sacral chakra is orange, a warm and expansive hue. Think of the beauty of orange fruit, the way colour combines with fragrance and taste to make it delicious. There is a joy in sacral chakra energy – not just the excitement and passion of sexual sharing, but also the timeless freedom of creative energy. When you truly express your creativity in whatever way suits you, time is somehow irrelevant. You pass into the Eternal Now, you are content, and know the joy of yourself.

Physically, this chakra connects with the sacrum, which is a triangle of fused bones connected to the large vertebrae of the lower back. This point is where the mobile bones of the spine join to a more fixed structure; it is particularly vulnerable to strain. Persistent lower back aches will benefit from sacral chakra support.

The element of the sacral chakra is water; it connects to the fluids of the male and female, to the waters of birth, as well as to tears and the emotions. It reminds us that all relationships are constantly flowing from one state to another, through positive times and challenges, always transforming and rebirthing into something new. This chakra helps us to understand change, and feel comfortable with it. It also connects us with each other, building all of our relationships; whatever we can achieve alone is enhanced when we work together.

Individually we are all also made up of both male and female energies – these can be expressed using the Chinese symbols of Yin (female, receptive, inner) and Yang (male, active, outer). The balance of these energies is maintained through the sacral chakra; so as well as helping our external relationships, this frequency also balances our inner relationships with ourselves.

SACRAL CHAKRA EMOTIONS

The sacral chakra links powerfully with the emotions, and human relationships are its testing ground. Jealousy, intolerance, irritation or envy are signs that the chakra is out of balance, If these difficult emotions are not tackled, they can lead to hormonal shifts in the body and problems such as impotence or emotional coldness.

Sacral chakra energy also links to the throat chakra, where the voice expresses our feelings. If our voice is emotionally blocked and we cannot say how we feel, there may be tension in the lower back and a lack of sexual energy. Communication is a role shared by these two chakras; the clearer we are when we speak, the easier our expression becomes in intimate relationships.

When the sacral chakra is in balance, we experience joy in ourselves and through being with others. We are ready to expand into relationships, to learn, grow and change. This chakra is also connected to the moon, waxing and waning throughout the year, governing the tides of the seas in an ever present symbol of flowing energy.

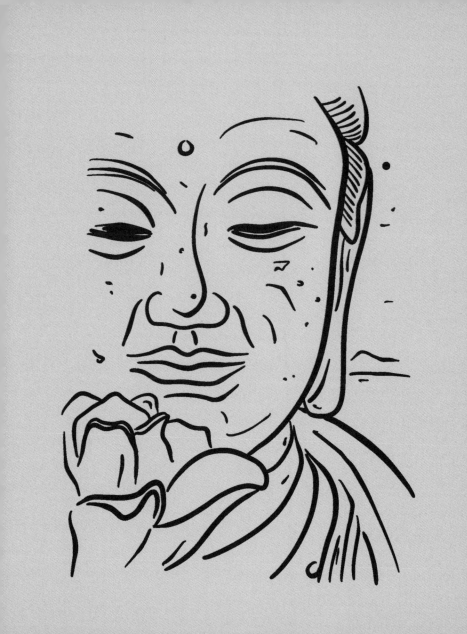

Every artist dips his brush in his own soul, and
paints his own nature into his pictures.

HENRY WARD BEECHER
(1814–1887)

Love many things, for therein lies the true strength,
and whosoever loves much performs much, and
can accomplish much, and what is done in love is
done well.

VINCENT VAN GOGH
(1853–1890)

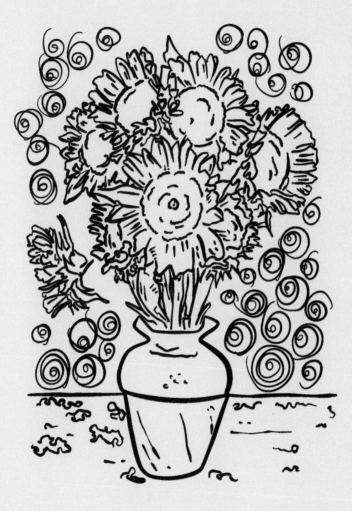

SACRAL CHAKRA YOGA

The Cat is a simple posture to energize the sacral chakra. If you have ever seen a cat flex and arch its back, and luxuriate in that stretch, you will have some idea of how good it feels to perform this movement. Only stretch as far as is comfortable – never strain. Three repetitions is enough to boost the sacral chakra. Regular use of this pose will also tone the lower back and digestive organs.

1 Kneel down on all fours, making sure your hands are directly in line with your shoulders, your arms straight and your knees parallel. Breathe regularly.

2 Exhale, and as you do so arch your back upwards as far as is comfortable, tilting your pelvis and pulling your stomach muscles upward. This really tones the lower abdomen and the lower back.

3 Inhale, and move the abdomen downwards, curving the lower back, lifting up your head to increase the stretch.

4 Return to the first position, breathe for a few moments then repeat the cycle again.

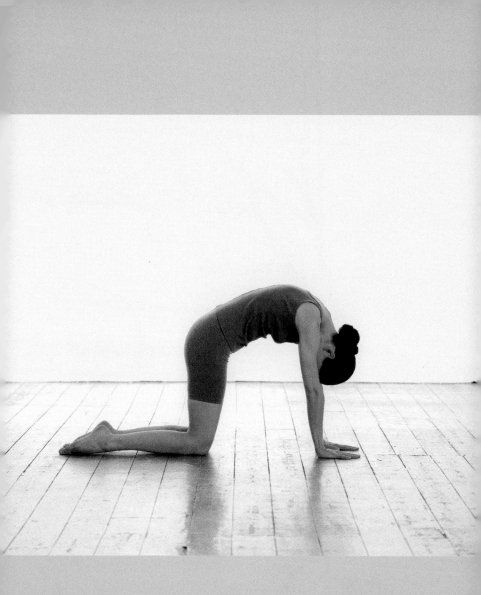

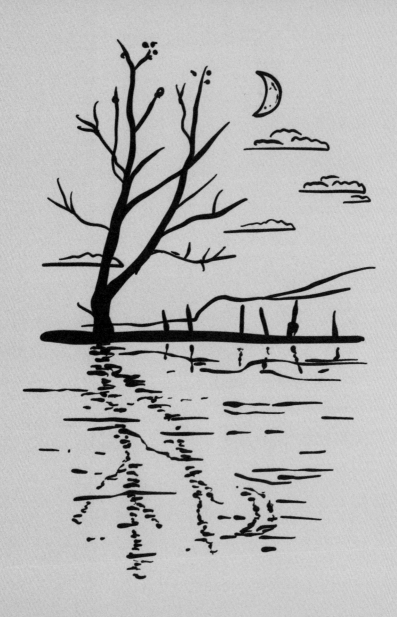

SACRAL CHAKRA VISUALIZATION

This exercise is helpful for releasing emotional sacral chakra issues. Sit comfortably in a chair or cross legged on the floor. Close your eyes, and breathe regularly.

Imagine you are sitting by an expanse of still water; either the sea or a lake. There is total peace and calm here, and a silvery glow lights the water's surface. As you watch, see the silver disc of a full moon rise slowly in the sky to sit above the water. Feel the effect of the gentle glow of the moonlight like a balm to your senses. Now notice a silvery pathway across the water toward the moon itself. You feel so full of light that you can take this path, your feet skimming across the surface of the water. As you approach the fullness of moon's glow, feel all negativity, sadness and anger dissolve away. The air is cool and gently fragrant, and you are at peace.

Feel your feet back on the ground, and you are standing back where you began, still observing the moon, as it dips below the horizon once more. Let your attention return gently to the present.

THE SOLAR PLEXUS CHAKRA

The solar plexus chakra is easiest to locate in the dip just under your ribcage at the front of the body. If you press your fingers inward here it can feel a little tender – this is quite normal because this area is also a major nerve plexus and therefore very sensitive. Named *manipura*, meaning "lustrous jewel", this chakra has a brilliant golden vibration like sunshine. It is a major source of energy for the whole body.

In spiritual terms, the solar plexus chakra is the place where the human being expresses ego – the demands and wishes of the lower self, linked to the will and drive to succeed. These are positive aspects of this chakra level, however in modern life the solar plexus is also vulnerable to manipulation, particularly by the media as the power of advertising drives and stimulates feelings such as greed and want. It is very important to keep the solar plexus chakra balanced at all times, especially if you live in an urban environment. The average journey to work in a town or city exposes you to at least 200 advertising messages that constantly work on your ego desires.

Positive solar plexus chakra influence on the ego is highly necessary; it encourages assertiveness rather than aggression, self-confidence rather than arrogance, healthy self-esteem rather than self-importance. This, in turn, improves and enhances our relationships at the sacral chakra level and clarifies our actions at the root chakra level. The lower three chakras work closely together and influence each other.

This chakra's element is fire, linked to the brilliant golden glow of its colour. Fire is fascinating; it can range from the small flickering glow of a candle flame to a vibrant blaze, or even a dazzling inferno. In many esoteric traditions fire is seen as cleansing, a way of disposing of old energy. One practical way to clear your solar plexus chakra of long-standing emotional negativity is to burn old diaries, papers and letters – do it in a sacred way, without resentment, let the fire dispose of them, and throw incense onto the glowing embers when you have finished. Performing this ceremony brings lightness and relief to your solar plexus chakra.

SOLAR PLEXUS EMOTIONS

The negative emotional level of the solar plexus chakra can resemble a stubborn angry child. Experiencing deep-rooted feelings that are almost too powerful to express, or a furious desire to control or manipulate others, are signs that this chakra is out of balance. To calm such explosive energy try taking ten deep breaths in and out, counting down from ten to one. This technique is a powerful self-help tool; you will feel its calming effect, and you will stop dissipating your energy. Of course, recognizing that you need to practise this technique is more than half the battle. People with stubborn egos tend to take some persuading because their strong will says that everyone else but them is at fault.

The demanding will of the lower self needs to be guided by the wisdom of the higher self. This your inner knowing, the "still small voice" inside your head that instinctively knows what is right. Listening to your higher self will help to rebalance the solar plexus chakra and calm the emotions.

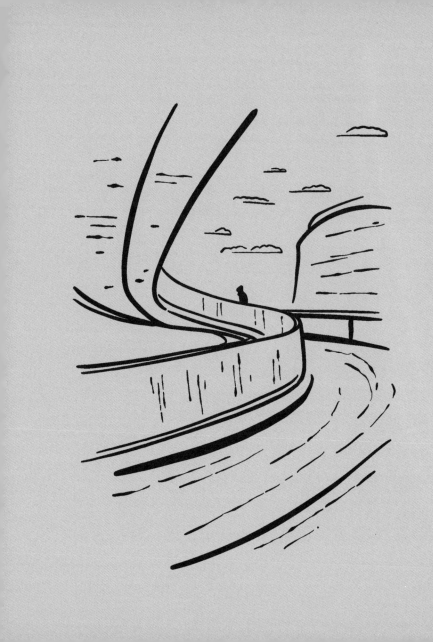

They can conquer who believe they can.

VIRGIL
(C70–C19BCE)

What lies behind us and what lies before us are tiny
matters compared to what lies within us.

RALPH WALDO EMERSON
(1803–1882)

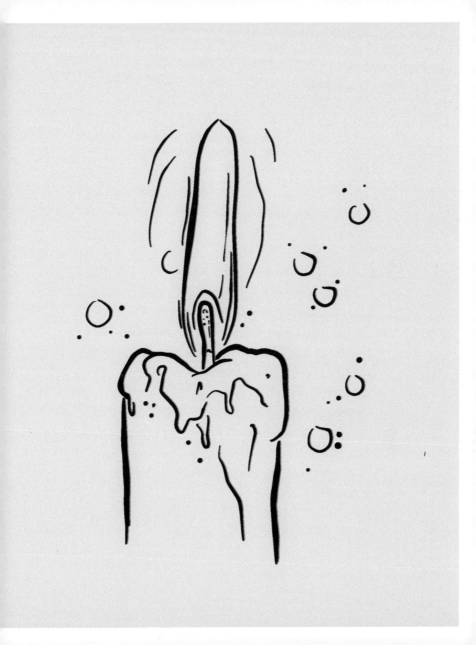

SOLAR PLEXUS CHAKRA YOGA

The solar plexus chakra can be calmed and rebalanced by using a yoga posture called the Sitting Forward Bend. Chakra centres are often worked by the "compression and release" of yoga postures, as is the case here.

1 Sit down on the floor with your legs stretched out in front of you, your back straight and your arms by your sides. Wriggle your hips slightly so you can feel your pelvic bones in contact with the floor.

2 Exhale, lift your arms forward and stretch down toward your feet from the level of your hips, keeping your back straight and pushing your chest forward so your body is folding in half.

3 Breathe easily, stretch down and hold your legs wherever is comfortable – perhaps your calves or your toes. Feel the muscles in your lower back and abdomen being worked, as well as the area of your solar plexus chakra.

4 To release, slowly work the hands back up the legs to support yourself to a sitting position.

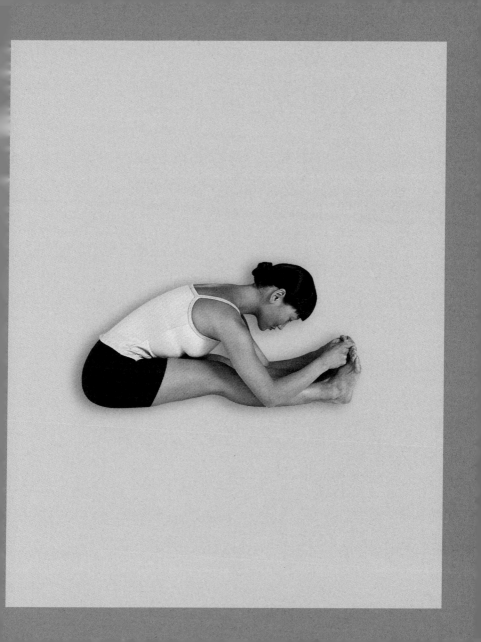

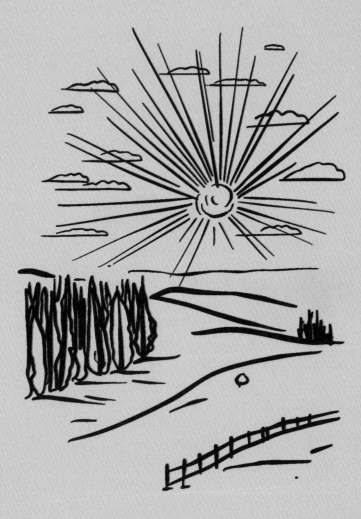

SOLAR PLEXUS CHAKRA VISUALIZATION

This exercise uses the image of the sun and golden light to revitalize and restore the solar plexus chakra. It is a good visualization to practise regularly if you live in an urban area as it cleanses and protects your energy field from negative influences. If you wish, light a candle before you start. Sit comfortably, hands in your lap.

Focus your mind on the area just below the ribcage where the solar plexus chakra is located. Breathe into this area, and as you do, see a ball of brilliant golden light glowing there. As you observe it, visualize the ball of light expanding in size until you are sitting within a globe of golden light that surrounds you and permeates you. Feel the cleansing, tingling and revitalizing effects of this golden light, which is connected to the sun. Feel it dissolving negative thoughts and emotions, leaving you full of light. Stay inside the globe for a few moments, and then see it begin to diminish in size, until it is back in place over your solar plexus chakra area. Breathe deeply, and notice how you feel in body and mind.

THE HEART CHAKRA

Of the seven colours of the rainbow (red, orange, yellow, green, blue, indigo and violet), green lies in the middle of the colour range. It is the colour of the heart chakra, which sits in the middle of the chest, balanced between the three lower chakras with their warmer physical energy and the three higher chakras, which have cooler tones and more cerebral frequencies. The heart chakra, in the middle, balances body and mind; it is a place of harmony and beauty. In nature we see the rich profusion of vibrant, lush green leaves reaching for the light of the sun. This energy of growth and expansion is the key to the heart chakra. Its element is air, which links it to the lungs and the expansion of the breath itself.

The Sanskrit name of the heart chakra is *anahata*, which means "unbeaten" or "unstruck", so-called because the heart is the location where love is felt and expressed, and very often it can feel struck and in pain. This is because human love is susceptible to influence by will – the influence of the solar plexus chakra

– trying to make things happen and then being hurt if they do not. If the heart chakra is "unbeaten" it is strong and radiates love from a higher level beyond the attachments and demands of the lower will. This is unconditional love. It simply exists, radiates, in an inexhaustible supply. It is love for all beings, all creatures, all that is and shall be.

Unconditional love is a state of being, not doing. Sometimes it can be a challenge, because as human beings we constantly have to balance the physical aspects of living and functioning in our bodies with the creative and inspirational aspects of our minds and spirits. The journey of life is a learning curve, and we are all subject to outside influences, to our desires, needs and wants. There is nothing wrong with any of these aspects of existence as long as none of them dominates. To be in a state of unconditional love is to know compassion, caring and tenderness for ourselves and those around us, without needing it back. Yet, wonderfully, if we give love unconditionally we will receive it in the same way. This is what Indian sages call the law of karma – "as you sow, so shall you reap".

HEART CHAKRA EMOTIONS

If your heart chakra is low in energy, then the feeling of love will be suppressed. You may suffer outbursts of bitterness or jealousy, especially if the solar plexus is involved and the will is demanding that desires be met. Closure of the heart chakra can lead to emotional withdrawal and loss of communication – here the problem may have immobilized the next chakra in the sequence, the throat chakra. The heart chakra has a vital part to play in creating emotional balance, so that love can be freely expressed and received.

Negative effects on heart chakra energy can show up in body language, such as the arms coiling around the body as extra protection. The arms and hands allow the heart chakra to physically express love through holding, touching, caressing and nurturing. If you feel your heart chakra is emotionally drained, go outside, stretch your arms wide and take some deep breaths. This is a simple way of rebalancing the heart chakra through its element of air, opening your body to give and receive love.

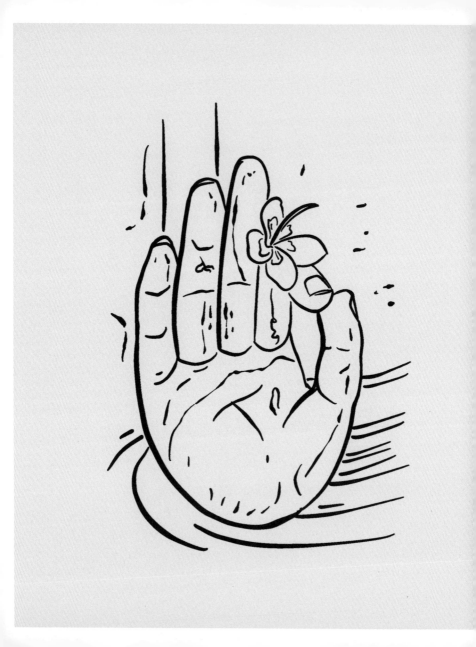

The little space within the heart is as great as the vast universe. The heavens and the earth are there, and the sun and the moon and the stars. Fire and lightning and winds are there, and all that is now and all that is not.

THE UPANISHADS
(8TH–4TH CENTURY BCE)

The only lasting beauty is the beauty of the heart.

RUMI
(1207–1273)

HEART CHAKRA YOGA

The Cobra is an excellent posture for opening the heart chakra. The curving of the spine pushes out the chest, re-energizing the location of the heart centre. This posture also tones the abdominal area and re-energizes the entire spinal column. Remember not to push yourself too far, especially if you are prone to back problems.

1 Lie face down on the floor with your legs together and your arms bent with your hands flat on the floor at shoulder level. Rest your forehead on the floor and breathe regularly for a moment.

2 Inhale, slowly lifting your forehead off the floor, and push up with your arms so that your chest is raised as high as you can go. Your arms will hold you steady. Keep your legs close together to maximize the stretch. Breathe in and out three times.

3 Slowly lower your arms so your upper body sinks back to the floor. Relax for a few moments. Feel the effects on your abdomen and chest. Repeat the posture if you wish.

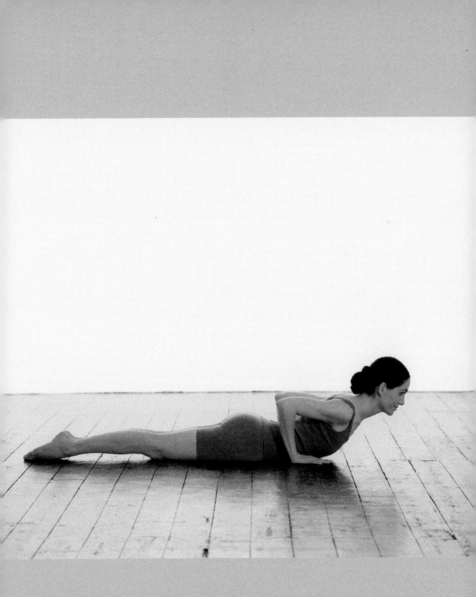

HEART CHAKRA VISUALIZATION

As well as the richness of green, another colour is often associated with the heart chakra as a symbol of unconditional love – pink. The best way to illustrate the role of these colours is in a visualization drawn from nature. Sit comfortably and relax, with your hands in your lap.

Imagine a small green shoot pushing up out of the ground, like a bulb in the springtime. The shoot is being drawn upwards by the warmth of the sun, and the more the sun shines, the taller the shoot grows. It sends tendrils outwards, and its buds open and spread into leaves, tilting themselves to catch the sun's rays so they can make food for the plant to grow strong, grow further. Now the plant is a rich profusion of green, expansive and vital. At its peak of growth, something new happens. A central bud forms that looks different. As you watch, the bud swells, opens and unfurls beautiful deep pink petals – a flower with a delicious soft sweet aroma. Enjoy the contrast of the rich green and soft pink colours and let this symbol relax and restore your heart chakra.

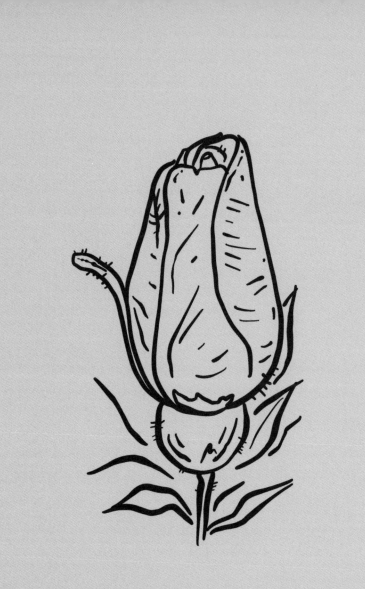

THE THROAT CHAKRA

The throat chakra lies in the base of the neck area in the dip where the collar bones meet. The Sanskrit name of the chakra is *vishuddha* which means "purification"; this links to the power of sound. Throat chakra energy is intimately concerned with the voice – with speaking, chanting and singing. The more the throat chakra is in balance, the purer our communication with each other. The mouth and throat are also where the breath enters the body on its way to inflate the lungs, and using the breath with the voice creates some of the most beautiful sounds a human being can make. The next time you hear an opera singer, think about this relationship – breath, voice, sound, song, harmony. The voice is a miraculous aspect of humanity, allowing communication and creativity as well as harmony through sound. The throat chakra gives energy to the voice.

The colour of the throat chakra is blue, which is a change of vibration into a much cooler tone, compared to the warm tones of the lower chakras. Colours like blue or purple are at the higher end of the colour spectrum and have a more subtle and soothing effect than the energizing reds, oranges and yellows at the lower end. The shade that links to the throat chakra is a deep sapphire. In medieval times, glass makers would pay vast sums for ground up lapis lazuli, a rare blue precious stone, to mix as a pigment for stained glass. The great Chartres Cathedral in France contains the famous Rose Window, which is full of sapphire blue glass, especially visible in the dim light of the interior. Illuminators of fine manuscripts in the medieval period also used ground lapis lazuli as a paint pigment to show the blue skies of heaven and the colour of the Virgin's robe.

The element of the throat chakra is ether. We have travelled from earth at the root chakra, through water at the sacral, fire at the solar plexus and air at the heart. Ether is the first level beyond the physical body. The energy of sound reverberates into this level and helps to purify the energetic blueprint of the body. This is why toning and chanting sacred sounds is such an effective way to heal, balance and support this chakra.

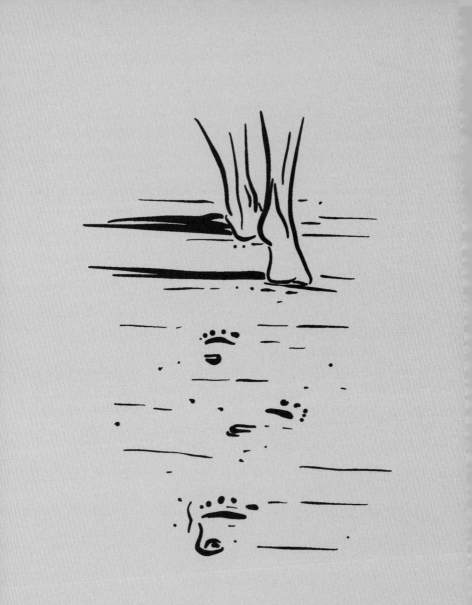

THROAT CHAKRA EMOTIONS

This chakra is deeply connected with self-expression. Each one of us is unique, we all have something to say. And our self-expression may take forms other than words; we may find a channel through a creative activity such as painting. We have the unique ability to translate inspiration into something concrete, and express this through the balanced medium of the throat chakra. The word "inspiration" is derived from the Latin *spirare*, meaning "to breathe". So the breath, drawn in through the throat chakra area, is vitally connected to throat chakra energy, which in turn feeds creative expression.

Often when we become stressed or emotionally frustrated, our throats feel tight and we feel as if we can't breathe. It is as if we are unable to express what we really want to say – or maybe we say something we will later regret. This causes stress to the throat chakra that will need to be released. To keep this chakra open and working well, it is important to be open and clear in the way you relate to others and express your own truth.

The one remains, the many change and pass;
Heaven's light forever shines, earth's shadows fly;
Life, like a dome of many-coloured glass, Stains the
white radiance of eternity.

PERCY BYSSHE SHELLEY
(1792–1822)

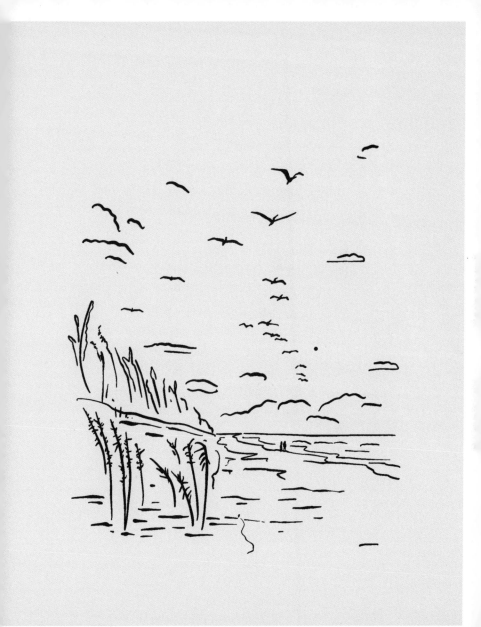

THROAT CHAKRA YOGA

The Plough posture helps to energize the throat chakra. It gives a deep stretch to the back as well as focusing energy around the throat area; when you release, you will feel lighter and freer in the body as a whole as well as in the neck and upper chest. If at first your toes don't reach the floor, keep practising – you will improve.

1 Lie down on your back with legs together and hands palm down by your sides.

2 Exhale, then, as you inhale, lift your legs and then your hips slowly up and over your head stretching your legs behind you, as low as you can, until the tips of your toes reach the floor. Support your back with your hands and breathe into the stretch for a minute or so.

3 To release, bend your knees and gently roll back out of the posture and lie quietly for a few moments.

4 Let your awareness go to your throat chakra area. Notice any feelings of energy, openness or tightness. Practice this posture to help harmonize throat chakra energy.

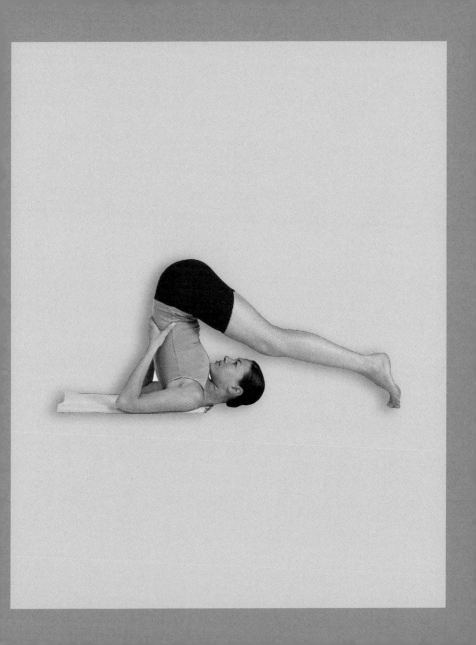

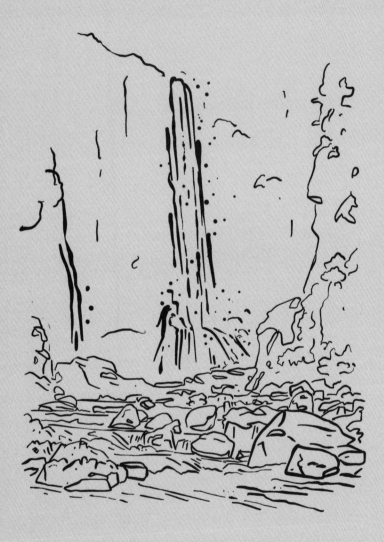

THROAT CHAKRA VISUALIZATION

Here we use the image of a waterfall to help the flow of energy through the throat chakra area. This visualization works to harmonize and calm you; imagining the movement of the water helps dislodge feelings of being stuck in any way. It will help release emotional constrictions in the throat area. Sit comfortably in a chair, hands resting on your knees. Breathe gently and regularly.

Visualize a waterfall plunging over the edge of a rocky outcrop, down into a plunge pool and on into a smooth flowing stream. Imagine the sound the water makes as it tumbles, see the swirling patterns in the deep blue plunge pool, feel the soft water vapour on your skin. Go into the water and stand under the waterfall; feel the power of the water pouring over your face and neck, and down your body. Feel this flowing energy pour through your throat chakra, cleansing blockages, moving away stuck feelings. Let them all go. When you are ready, step out of the water and onto the bank. Relax, breathe, and feel the sense of openness in your throat chakra.

THE THIRD EYE CHAKRA

The third eye chakra sits between the eyebrows, and is associated with the colour indigo, the deep purplish blue of the night sky. Its Sanskrit name is *ajna*, meaning "to perceive"; this chakra is intimately associated with intuition, the "sixth sense" instinctive knowing that is mysterious but somehow right. This is the also the sixth chakra in the frequency pattern that starts at the root and culminates in the seventh chakra at the crown.

The third eye chakra is the home of intelligence. This can be physical, emotional, mental or spiritual – it does not just mean "being clever". We have the capacity, via our chakras, to know our physical bodies, to relate to our feelings, to understand our world and to be inspired spiritually – these are all elements of our intelligence. The third eye is where these elements combine to give us a complete perception of ourselves and the world around us. This creates the conditions for intuition – the creative leap into the unknown. Human evolution would not have happened without such leaps. Today we face big questions about ourselves as a species, how we are populating the planet and using up its resources. The answers lie in the exercise of our full awareness and intelligence.

The ancient mantra or sacred sound OM helps to open the third eye chakra and stimulate the energy of awareness and creativity. OM is a sound that connects all things, from the tiniest atom within you to the vastness of the stars. At this chakra we are moving beyond the physical body into the realm of light – this light is the subtle element associated with the third eye. Chanting OM brings the light of the cosmos into the physical body.

Working with the third eye and crown chakras is best begun when the lower chakras are a well-balanced foundation and any major blocks there have been cleared. This creates a solid, stable framework for spiritual expansion. Your intuition will tell you if this is the right time for you to expand these higher frequencies; but be on guard against the negative ego will of the solar plexus chakra wanting it all too soon. Be patient with yourself; this a lifetime of work. The flower does not force its journey to the sun, it grows and unfolds in its own time.

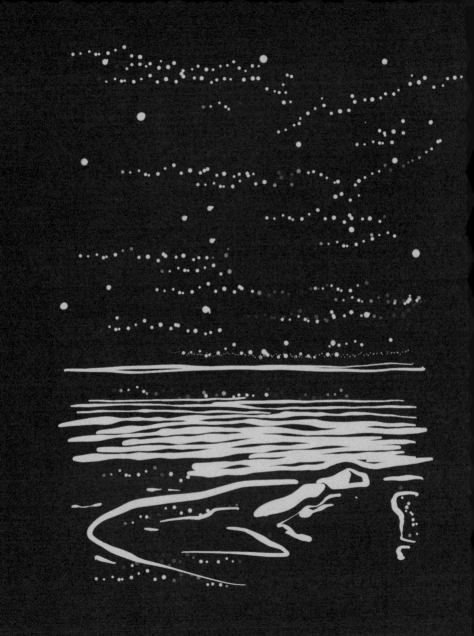

THIRD EYE CHAKRA EMOTIONS

Many issues arising in the third eye chakra energy frequency arise because one or more of the lower chakras are out of balance and are affecting it. For example, solar plexus tension, frustration and demands can create mental tension leading to headaches and migraines in the third eye area. Another example is sexual tension or coldness in the sacrum and root chakras, which can also lead to migraines. This is why the lower chakra issues need to be cleared to allow the third eye to function well.

Mental states such as anxiety, fear, confusion and insecurity also show there is low energy in the third eye chakra. It is important to ground the whole system using root chakra techniques before working specifically with the third eye. A wonderful way to do this is to go outside on a clear night and just look at the stars, sitting in the deep indigo of the night sky. As the colour of the third eye chakra bathes your senses, feel your feet very firmly rooted to the ground. This helps you to feel centred, stable and strong within yourself.

It's not what you look at that matters,

it's what you see.

HENRY DAVID THOREAU
(1817-1862)

We are such stuff as dreams are made of, and our

little lives are rounded with a sleep.

WILLIAM SHAKESPEARE
(1564–1616)

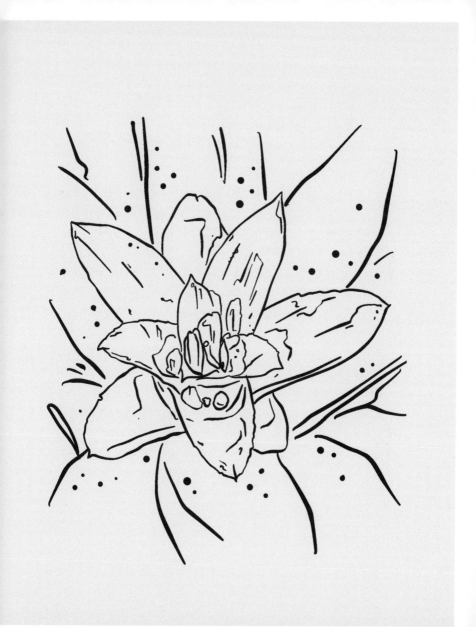

THIRD EYE CHAKRA YOGA

This wonderful yoga posture, called the Fish, works on the spine, chest, throat and third eye chakra. It is a deep stretch, so should only be attempted after the body has been loosened using a few of the previous yoga postures.

1 Lie flat on your back on the floor with your arms by your sides and your feet together. Breathe deeply a few times. Slide your hands, palms down, under your buttocks, reaching down your thighs as far as possible so your arms are straight.

2 Now inhale, press down on your elbows and lift your chest up off the floor so your lower back is arched. Your arms and hands are your support.

3 Exhale and let the top of your head gently touch the floor without leaning on it. Breathe regularly and feel the stretch in your chest, lungs, abdomen, back and neck, as well as the effect on the third eye chakra.

4 To release, lift the head, place it back on the floor and lower the arms slowly.

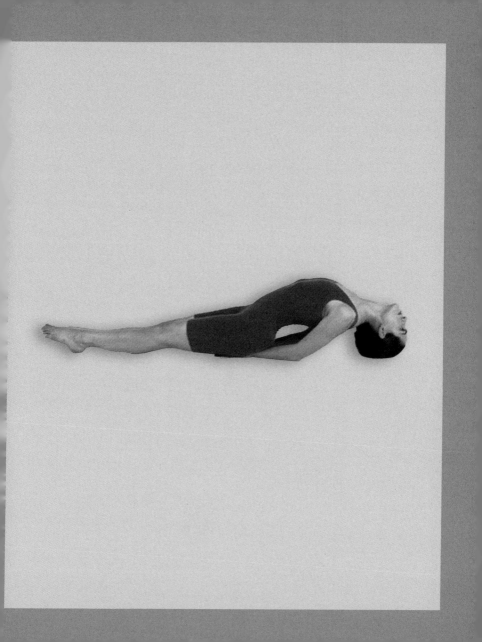

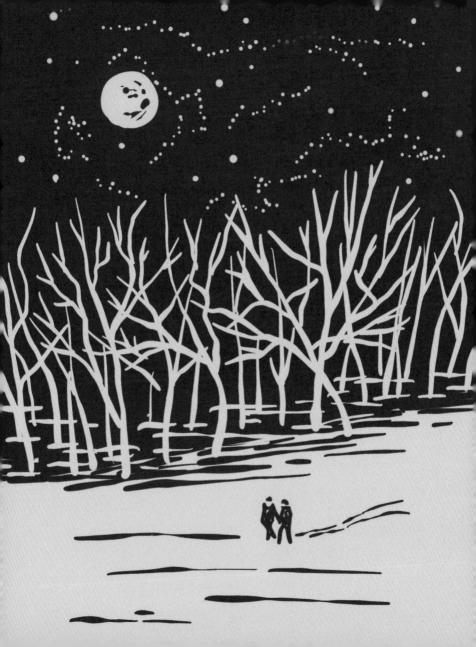

THIRD EYE CHAKRA VISUALIZATION

In many traditions the night sky is seen as a map beyond the earth to realms of deep wisdom. Somewhere in the sky is your star, the place that is your spiritual home. Finding this place will enhance the intuition which comes to you from the third eye chakra. Light a candle if you wish. Sit quietly and relax.

Visualize a night sky, deep purple-blue, scattered with millions of diamond bright stars. Feel a cool sense of peace as you contemplate the infinite space. Let your third eye chakra be calm, open, receptive. As your vision travels over the image of the sky, there is one star that draws you. Focus on this point of light and see it grow as if you are moving toward it. Notice what kind of star it is, the colour it radiates, if it has rings. You may even perceive it within a galaxy, a vast spiral of stars. However it appears, it is a heavenly beacon that only you recognize. Sit and be with your star, noticing what information, impressions or feelings arise. Breathe, and stretch your feet and hands to bring your awareness back to earth.

THE CROWN CHAKRA

The crown chakra sits at the very top of the head. In a newborn baby, the skull bones here are still unfused, and the ancient traditions of India and the East believe this is to maintain the connection to Divine Source for a short while until the spirit has grounded into the body of the newborn human. They teach that conception and birth are not simply biological functions, but arise from the blending of male and female energies combined with a spark from the Divine Source to create a new being.

This link to the source of creation is maintained via the crown chakra. Its colour is violet or white and its Sanskrit name is *sahasrara*, meaning "thousand petalled lotus". The lotus flower is sacred in Indian tradition; it has roots in mud at the bottom of a lake, symbolizing the weight of the material realm, then its stem travels up toward the light through water, symbolizing the realm of emotion. At the water's surface the leaves spread out as a platform to sunlight in the realm of air, and finally the flower forms, opening a perfect array of petals, releasing an exquisite fragrance into the subtle etheric realms. The lotus echoes the map of the chakras in each of us.

The crown chakra is your connection to whatever you believe to be spirit, Source, the divine spark of creation. Even if you think you are not a spiritual person, you still have this energy level within you. Do not be confused by words. The subtlety of the crown chakra is beyond them. You can find spirit in many places – from the most glorious of cathedrals to a raindrop gleaming on a blade of grass in the morning sun. It is whatever speaks to you of connection and love beyond everyday existence.

At the root chakra we are concerned with survival, and at the sacral chakra with creativity and reproductive energy. At the solar plexus chakra we find the powerful will, and at the heart, expansion into love. At the throat chakra feelings and thoughts find expression and at the third eye chakra our intuition opens. At the crown we experience our own connection with Source; if we have prepared the way and cleared away personal blocks, we experience spirit while still in the body. This is what the ancients called "enlightenment".

CROWN CHAKRA EMOTIONS

Crown chakra energy is the highest frequency in the body. It is linked to pineal gland function and to conditions such as depression or Seasonal Affective Disorder. It is also likely that children diagnosed with hyperactivity or ADHD have some kind of crown chakra imbalance.

Crown chakra issues can also manifest as challenging psychological conditions such as dementia, schizophrenia and other severe mental illnesses, where concepts of reality are shattered and uncertain, leading to irrational behaviour, confusion and great vulnerability. Therapies using the senses as a means of communication can help people with these conditions. Touch, sound, colour and aromas all help to rebalance the chakra system, bringing grounding and a better sense of connection to the world.

To rebalance your crown chakra, lie down and place your hands parallel on the top of your head, fingers toward the back of your skull. Stay like this for several minutes. You may feel pulsations under your hands. Wait for an even rhythm; this brings peace and calm.

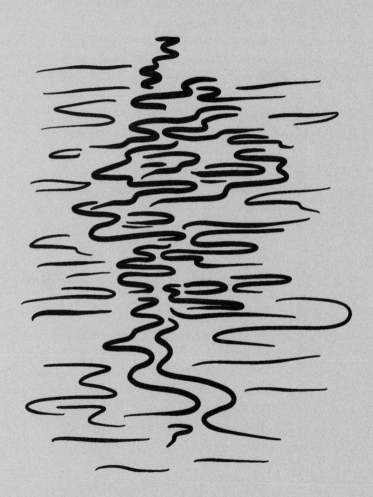

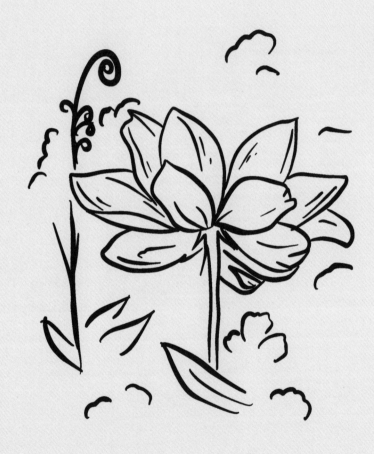

Higher than the senses are the objects of sense.
Higher than the objects of sense is the mind;
And higher than the mind is the intellect.
Higher than the intellect is the Great Self.
Higher than the Great Self is the Unmanifest.
Higher than the Unmanifest is the Person.
Higher than the Person there is nothing at all.
That is the goal. That is the highest course.

KATHA UPANISHAD
(1400–800BCE)

CROWN CHAKRA YOGA

The most common yoga posture associated with the crown chakra is the Lotus position. It can be difficult to achieve this pose if you are not supple, so the variation shown here is the Half Lotus, which is easier to perform. This posture encourages a straight spine. Practise it after you have tried some of the others suggested earlier, as the higher chakra frequencies should be opened only when the lower ones are balanced.

1 Sit on the floor with your legs stretched out in front of you in a V shape, your spine very straight.

2 Bend your right leg and bring the foot to rest as high as you can up the left thigh.

3 Bend your left leg and slide your left foot under your right thigh.

4 Rest your hands on your knees, close your eyes, breathe deeply, and visualize violet light at your crown chakra.

5 Stay in the pose as long as is comfortable – maybe only a few minutes at first. It is an ideal asana for meditation.

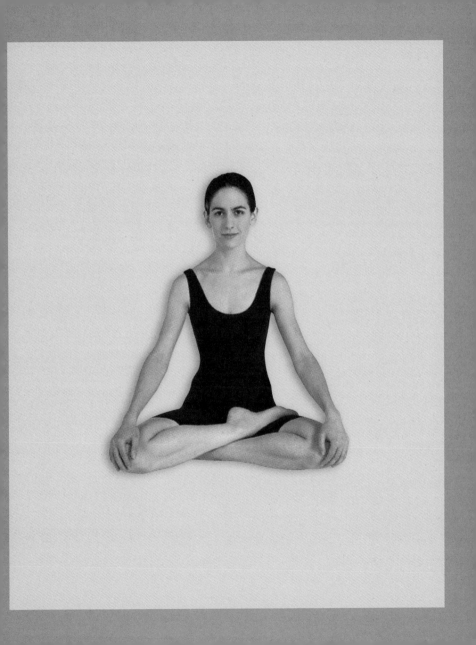

CROWN CHAKRA VISUALIZATION

This simple but powerful exercise uses the brilliant light of a diamond, which reflects all the colours in the rainbow spectrum. Ground yourself before you start; try walking around barefooted in your home for a few minutes, feeling the difference between carpet, lino or ceramic floors under your feet. This helps to centre you. Light a candle if you wish. Sit in the half lotus posture.

Visualize a beautifully faceted, tear-drop shaped diamond in front of your eyes. Notice all the colours that it reflects – from fiery reds and oranges or brillant gold to greens, blues and purples. As you gaze at the diamond all the colours merge and become a brilliant white light, crystal clear. Now imagine the diamond placed above your crown chakra, so this white light can shine down through it and all the other chakras, energizing them; and that light can travel all the way into the earth itself. Feel yourself centred and bathed in the white light of the cosmos. Take a few deep breaths and uncross your legs, stretching them, to return to the present moment.

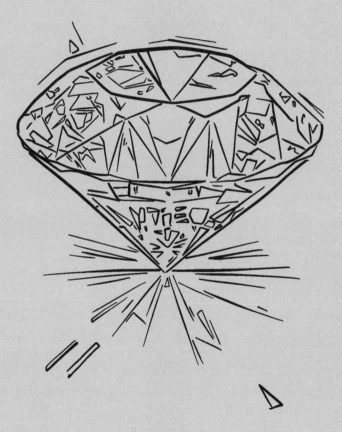

CHAPTER

The Whole System

Having explored all seven chakras individually, we move onto exercises which can balance the whole chakra system. This kind of work balances you generally. It is not as intense as focusing attention on a particular chakra level but benefits you greatly on an integrated level. You could also use these exercises to begin with, if you are still unsure where to start your chakra exploration.

We shall be working with colour, sound, aromas and crystals. Each of these healing modes can have greatly beneficial effects on chakra energies. They work on different sensory levels – sight, sound, smell and touch. The suggested

FOUR...

exercises are all drawn from highly developed healing methods – colour therapy, toning and sound therapy, Ayurveda, aromatherapy, and crystal healing. Each of these approaches is an in-depth and complex tool in itself, offering far more than we can cover in these pages. Use these ideas as a starting point. If you feel an affinity with one particular approach, explore it further. There are many excellent books available to help you do this.

If you are a newcomer to any of these therapeutic approaches, follow my instructions especially carefully. However, everything I have suggested is simple and safe, and should result in a balancing effect across your whole chakra system.

SEVEN CHAKRA COLOUR MEDITATION

This exercise takes you through the whole colour spectrum and gently balances all your chakras. It is a lovely visualization to use whenever you need to feel refreshed and revitalized. Light a candle if you wish and sit comfortably in a chair, hands relaxed on your lap.

Take a few deep breaths to relax. Focus on your spine; feel where it touches the chair. Concentrate on the root chakra, and visualize a ball of deep red. Move up and focus on the sacral chakra, and see a ball of glowing orange. Then go higher, to the solar plexus chakra, and see a ball of golden light. Focus on the heart chakra, and visualize a ball of vibrant green. Move to the throat chakra and see a ball of sapphire-blue light. Then go to the third eye chakra, and see a ball of deep indigo. Finally, move to the crown chakra, and see a ball of violet light.

Relax and bathe in the seven colours. After a few moments see the crown chakra ball shrink to a point of violet light; move down and see each chakra close in this way. This keeps the chakras receptive but not overactive.

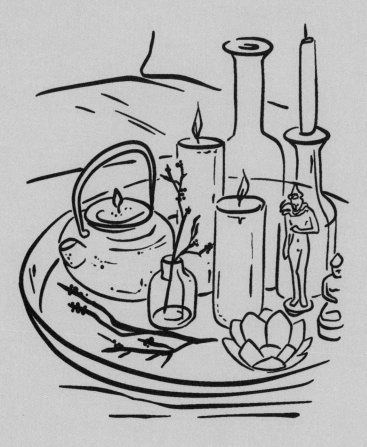

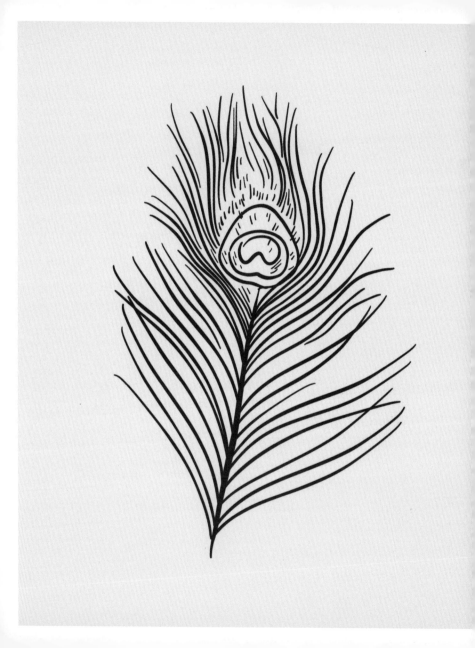

Nature does not hurry, yet everything
is accomplished.

LAO-TZU
(C.604–C.531BCE)

Whatever is in any way beautiful has its source of
beauty in itself, and is complete in itself.

MARCUS AURELIUS
(121–180CE)

SEVEN CHAKRA TONING EXERCISE

The practice of chanting or toning mantras heals and balances all the chakras. Vowel sounds are universally pure because the mouth is open when they are made; consonants close the vowels, bringing them to earth. The mantras below are traditional variations of consonants around the sound "A" (ahh), culminating in "M" (mmm), a humming sound. Each chakra also corresponds to a note in a simple musical scale: try picking this out using a keyboard or a recorder to get the pitch.

Tone each mantra once in sequence, and feel the difference between the sounds. For the root chakra, sound LAM (musical note C); for the sacral, VAM (note D); for the solar plexus, RAM (note E); for the heart, YAM (note F); for the throat, HAM (note G); for the third eye, OM (note A); and for the crown chakra, sound AUM (note B).

To begin with, write a list of the mantras to help you get the sequence correct. If you find that toning a scale is difficult, choose a note that is comfortable for you and keep the same pitch for all the mantras.

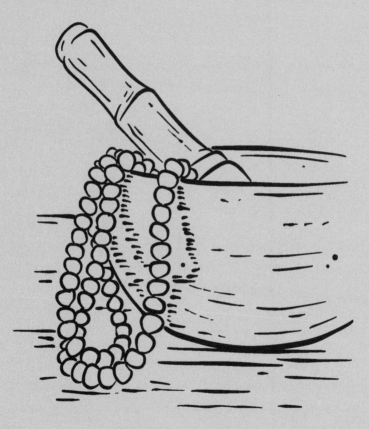

ESSENTIAL OILS AND THE CHAKRAS

Essential oils are highly concentrated fragrances extracted from plants. They have been used in traditional Indian medicine for centuries as subtle agents of healing, especially when applied directly to energy sites such as the seven major chakras. They are also used in aromatherapy, where they are blended into a vegetable carrier oil and massaged over the whole body to bring relaxation and well-being. Diluting essential oils to the exact specifications of a particular blend is vital to prevent any skin irritation or adverse reaction, and they are for external use only – never swallow them.

To use essential oils to balance chakra energies, you need to make a blend and apply it directly over the chakra site. This is not massage in the aromatherapy sense, it is a more Ayurvedic (traditional Indian medicine) approach. The blend is massaged into the skin in a clockwise circular motion at the location of the chakra over a small area about the size of an apple, for about three minutes. The effect of this will be very subtle. The chakra location is like a gateway that allows the healing properties of the essential oils to penetrate the body.

When you have decided which chakra to work on, make up the appropriate essential oil blend from the list on page 118 to support, balance and harmonize your chosen chakra. For each blend, you will need 4 tsps (20ml) of organic sunflower oil as a carrier, poured into a small, clean, dark-glass bottle. Add the essential oil drops exactly as indicated; then shake the mixture. To apply the blend, massage about half a teaspoon of oil onto the chakra area with firm but not hard pressure, in a clockwise direction. Work for three minutes then relax. You can choose to work on the front or the back of the body. Apply your chakra blend after a bath or shower, once or twice a day as you wish. After a few days, you should feel a difference in that chakra area. If you feel you need to work on a new level, make up the appropriate blend, and apply it in the same way.

For the crown chakra, make up the blend in 4 tsps (20ml) unfragranced shampoo, so you can massage it into your scalp and then use it to wash your hair too.

Essential oil blends for the chakras

Remember, each combination is blended in a carrier of 4 tsps organic sunflower oil. Add the essential oils to the carrier, shake the bottle and then the blend is ready.

✤ **Root chakra** 2 drops vetiver, 2 drops ginger: an earthy and deeply warming aroma, very grounding.

✤ **Sacral chakra** 2 drops sandalwood, 2 drops sweet orange: a woody and softly citrus aroma that is opening and cheering.

✤ **Solar plexus chakra** 2 drops grapefruit, 2 drops fennel: a zesty and slightly aniseed aroma, purifying and bright.

✤ **Heart chakra** 2 drops rose otto, 2 drops cardamom: a rich, sweet and spicy aroma, expanding and warming.

✤ **Throat chakra** 2 drops Roman chamomile, 2 drops manuka: a soft, slightly fruity and gently spicy aroma, opening and soothing.

✤ **Third eye chakra** 2 drops frankincense, 2 drops sweet basil: an uplifting, resiny aroma, expanding perception.

✤ **Crown chakra** 2 drops neroli, 2 drops rosewood: an exquisitely soft, gentle and expansive aroma.

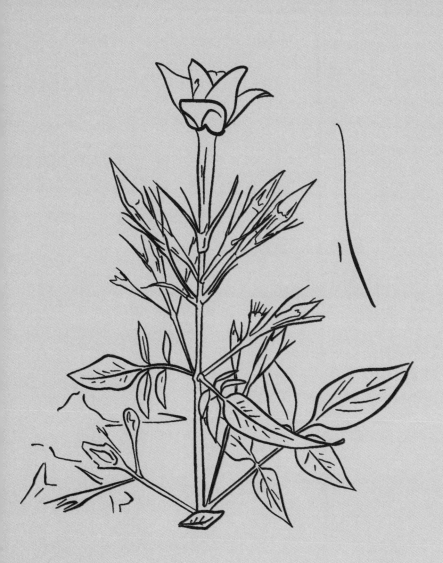

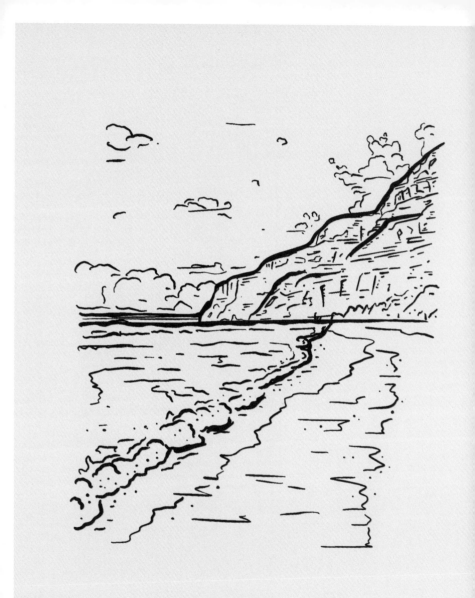

I offer you peace.

I offer you love.

I offer you friendship.

I see your beauty.

I hear your need.

I feel your feelings.

My wisdom flows from the Highest Source.

I salute that Source in you.

Let us work together for unity and love.

MAHATMA GANDHI
(1869–1948)

CRYSTALS AND THE CHAKRAS

Crystals are amazing combinations of minerals that respond to particular chemical reactions of warming and cooling within the earth's crust to produce geometric formations in stunning colours. They have been discovered and mined by humankind since the dawn of time. Ancient cultures worldwide made links between these stones and the realm of spirit, wearing them as sacred symbols or using them in healing practices.

The ancient Egyptians were particularly skilled at making ritual jewellery, such as royal crowns and collars of gold inlaid with blue lapis lazuli, red carnelian and black onyx. The Aztecs astounded the Spanish invaders with the enormous emeralds they wore as their most sacred stones. Indian potentates would be literally covered in gems from head to foot, and even had them sewn into their clothing. These ancient cultures used gems and crystals to show power and wealth, but they were also aware of the subtle and healing aspects of each stone and why it was necessary to place them in certain ways.

Do you ever wonder why you choose particular jewellery on a particular day? It could be that instinctively you are choosing a stone to energize a chakra. Garnet, bloodstone and hematite correspond to the root chakra and reflect this chakra's red colour. Amber, carnelian and coral energize the sacral chakra and reflect warm orange tones. The wonderful golden stones of citrine (a sparkling yellow quartz), gold tiger's eye and gold topaz clear and cleanse the solar plexus chakra. Aventurine and emerald are green stones that help support the expansive heart chakra. Rose quartz is also linked to this area as it reflects the pink of unconditional love. The sky-blue crystal celestite, the blue-green turquoise and the soft blue lace agate all help to soothe the throat chakra. Lapis lazuli, sapphire and amethyst all correspond to the third eye chakra. These stones shine with varying tones of deep blue or purple; these are softer in lapis lazuli and amethyst, and brilliant in sapphire. Clear quartz and diamonds support the crown chakra. This chakra reflects a dazzling white colour, as seen in these beautiful stones.

A crystal healing exercise for the chakras

This exercise uses a simple crystal healing layout to balance the chakras. You will need to work with a friend and require eight crystals in all, one each of bloodstone, carnelian, citrine, aventurine, rose quartz, blue lace agate, amethyst and clear quartz. These can be small "tumble" stones, available from crystal suppliers. Rinse them under cold water before you use them to cleanse them.

The person receiving the treatment needs to lie comfortably on the floor, with their head on a pillow, and be covered with a clean white sheet. The person giving the treatment should place the crystals on the body as follows: bloodstone on the lower abdomen; carnelian over the navel, citrine over the solar plexus; aventurine and rose quartz over the centre of the chest; blue lace agate at the throat; amethyst on the forehead; and clear quartz on the floor over the top of the head. Let the recipient rest for about ten minutes bathed in the crystal energies. Then remove the crystals and run them under cold water to cleanse them again. Relax and discuss how the exercise felt, then swap places with your friend and repeat.

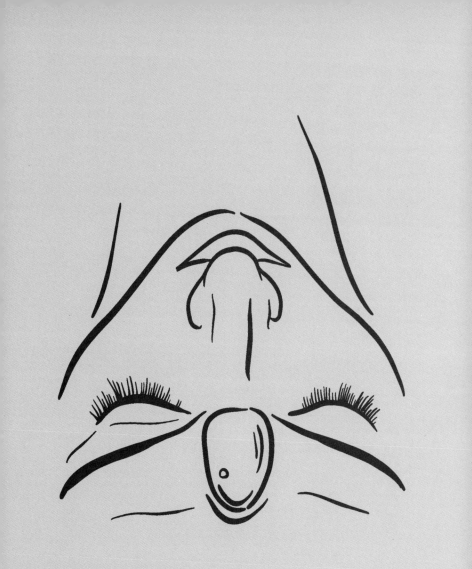